KETO DIET QUICK AND EASY RECIPES 2021/22

This cookbook was created to achieve the goal of losing weight in the shortest time possible, I propose a series of recipes Easy Quick to prepare the famous Keto Diet, eat healthy and get back in shape.

Gianni Stefanelli

KETO DIET QUICK AND EASY RECIPES 2021/22

Gianni Stefanelli

THIS COOKBOOK WAS CREATED TO ACHIEVE THE GOAL OF LOSING WEIGHT IN THE SHORTEST TIME POSSIBLE, I PROPOSE A SERIES OF RECIPES EASY QUICK TO PREPARE THE FAMOUS KETO DIET, EAT HEALTHY AND GET BACK IN SHAPE.

Table Of Contents

The information in the following pages is broadly considered a truthful and accurate account of facts and as such, any inattention, use, or misuse of the information in question by the reader will render any resulting actions solely under their purview. There are no scenarios in which the publisher or the original author of this work can be in any fashion deemed liable for any hardship or damages that may befall them after undertaking information described herein.

Additionally, the information in the following pages is intended only for informational purposes and should thus be thought of as universal. As befitting its nature, it is presented without assurance regarding its prolonged validity or interim quality. Trademarks that are mentioned are done without written consent and can in no way be considered an endorsement from the trademark holder.

☆ 55% OFF for BookStore NOW at $ 24,95 instead of $ 35,95! ☆

It is known that the recipes of the Ketogenic diet

are not really simple; in fact, it is this type of diet is

not easy to follow.

That's why I created this book,

a series of recipes that will allow you to prepare

your dishes in a simple and fast way.

Buy is NOW and let your Customers get addicted to this amazing book!

Introduction

The ketogenic diet: what is it?

The ketogenic diet is a protein diet, however rich in protein.

It allows a weight loss of about 2 kg per week and has its origins as a therapy against epilepsy because it was found that in epileptic patients, during periods of fasting, seizures were greatly reduced.

The ketogenic diet, almost devoid of carbohydrates, induces in the body the same mechanisms of fasting, stimulating the destruction of fats to produce carbohydrates - indispensable to the human body (about 200 grams of glucose per day) - but at the same time provides nutrients such as protein and (little) fiber.

The conversion of carbohydrates thus carried out, however, produces waste substances called ketone bodies, which are very difficult to dispose of for the liver and kidneys, resulting in toxic in large quantities.

Allowed foods of the ketogenic diet categories of foods allowed in the ketogenic diet fats: condiments such as olive oil, butter, soybean oil, sesame oil, lard, real foods such as those derived from cheeses that are rich in fat and protein but low in carbohydrates such as dairy flakes or mozzarella or ricotta. Mayonnaise can also be consumed;

proteins: eggs; meat, game, steak, lamb, chicken, sausage, hamburger, turkey, preserved meats such as speck, ham, bacon, bresaola, smoked meat. Fish, shellfish, salmon, tuna, herring, lobster, shrimp, anchovies;

vegetables (maximum 500 grams per day) low in carbohydrates (zucchini, asparagus, mushrooms, broccoli);

a good amount of supplements to compensate for deficiencies: including milk protein (to prevent the destruction of proteins due to the reduction of carbohydrates); peptide Glutamine (counteracts the nitrogenous waste produced in the metabolism of proteins); branched-chain amino acids (to prevent the body from using muscle protein); L-carnitine (to help the ketogenic metabolism); mineral salts (which are not provided by the diet, poor in fruit);

water: at least 2 liters per day, or unsweetened tea or herbal tea; Dried fruits Salt, pepper, mustard

It is known that the recipes of the Ketogenic diet are not really simple; in fact, it is this type of diet is not easy to follow. That's why I created this book, a series of recipes that will allow you to prepare your dishes in a simple and fast way.

EASY BREAKFAST

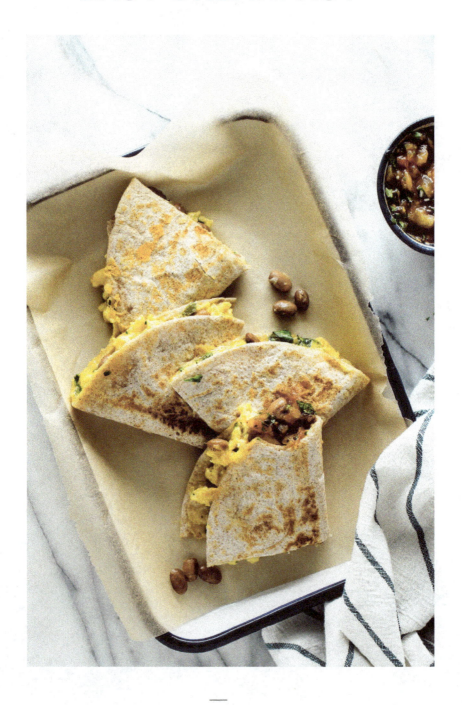

Naan Bread And Butter

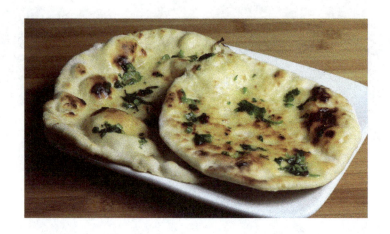

Servings: 6
Prep time: 10 min

INGREDIENTS:

7 tablespoons coconut oil
¾ cup coconut flour
2 tablespoons psyllium powder
½ teaspoon baking powder
Salt to the taste
2 cups hot water
Some coconut oil for frying
2 garlic cloves, minced
3.5 ounces ghee

DESCRIPTION:

In a bowl, mix coconut flour with baking powder, salt and psyllium powder and stir.

Add 7 tablespoons coconut oil and the hot water and start kneading your dough.

Leave aside for 5 minutes, divide into 6 balls and flatten them on a working surface.

Heat up a pan with some coconut oil over medium-high heat, add naan bread to the pan, fry them until they are golden and transfer them to a plate.

Warm-up a pan with the ghee over medium-high heat, add garlic, salt and pepper, stir and cook for 2 minutes.

Brush naan bread with this mix and pour the rest into a bowl.

Serve in the morning.

Nutrition Value:
calories 146, fat 9,8, fiber 2, carbs 3,9, protein 5

Breakfast Salad In A Jar

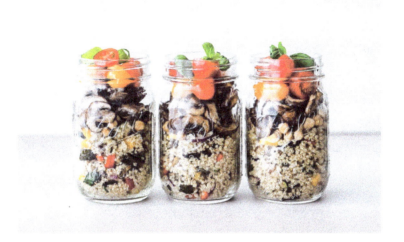

Servings: 6
Prep time: 10 min

INGREDIENTS:

1-ounce favorite greens
1-ounce red bell pepper, chopped
1-ounce cherry tomatoes, halved
4 ounces rotisserie chicken, roughly chopped
4 tablespoons extra virgin olive oil
½ scallion, chopped
1-ounce cucumber, chopped
Salt and black pepper to the taste

DESCRIPTION:

In a bowl, mix greens with bell pepper, tomatoes,
scallion, cucumber, salt, pepper and olive oil and toss
to coat well.
Transfer this to a jar, top with chicken pieces and
serve for breakfast.

Nutrition Value:
calories 185, fat 12, fiber 4, carbs 7, protein 19

Feta Omelet

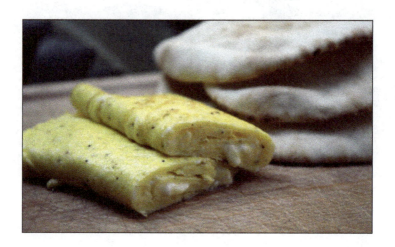

Servings: 4
Prep time: 10 min

INGREDIENTS:

3 eggs
1 tablespoon ghee
1 ounce feta cheese, crumbled
1 tablespoon heavy cream
1 tablespoon jarred pesto
Salt and black pepper to the taste

DESCRIPTION:

In a bowl, mix eggs with heavy cream, salt and pepper and whisk well.

Heat up a pan with the ghee over medium high heat, add whisked eggs, spread into the pan and cook your omelet until it's fluffy.

Sprinkle cheese and spread pesto on your omelet, fold in half, cover pan and cook for 5 minutes more.

Transfer omelet to a plate and serve.

Nutrition Value:
calories 506, fat 43, fiber 6,9, carbs 3,6, protein 34

Chicken Quiche

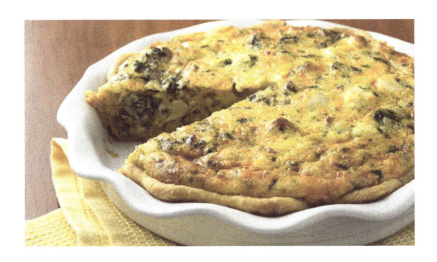

Servings: 4
Prep time: 10 min

INGREDIENTS:

7 eggs
2 cups almond flour
2 tablespoons coconut oil
Salt and black pepper to the taste
2 zucchinis, grated
½ cup heavy cream
1 teaspoon fennel seeds
1 teaspoon oregano, dried
1 pound chicken meat, ground

DESCRIPTION:

In your food processor, blend almond flour with a pinch of salt.

Add one egg and coconut oil and blend well.

Place dough in a greased pie pan and press well on the bottom.

Heat up a pan over medium heat, add chicken meat, brown for a couple of minutes, take off heat and leave aside.

In a bowl, mix six eggs with salt, pepper, oregano, cream and fennel seeds and whisk well.

Add chicken meat and stir again.

Pour this into pie crust, spread, introduce in the oven at 350 degrees F and bake for 40 minutes.

Leave the pie to cool down a bit before slicing and serving it for breakfast!

Nutrition Value:
calories 321, fat 25, fiber 5, carbs 4, protein 19

Breakfast French Toast

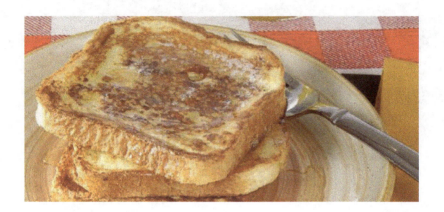

Servings: 4
Prep time: 40 min

INGREDIENTS:

1 cup whey protein
12 egg whites
4 ounces cream cheese
For the French toast:
1 teaspoon vanilla
½ cup coconut milk
2 eggs
1 teaspoon cinnamon, ground
½ cup ghee, melted
½ cup almond milk
½ cup swerve

DESCRIPTION:

In a bowl, mix egg whites with your mixer for a few minutes.

Add protein and stir gently.

Add cream cheese and stir again.

Pour this into 2 greased bread pans, introduce in the oven at 325 degrees F and bake for 45 minutes.

Leave breads to cool down and slice them into 18 pieces.

In a bowl, mix 2 eggs with vanilla, cinnamon and coconut milk and whisk well.

Dip bread slices in this mix.

Heat up a pan with some coconut oil over medium heat, add bread slices, cook until they are golden on each side and divide between plates.

Heat up a pan with the ghee over high heat, add almond milk and heat up well.

Add swerve, stir and take off heat.

Leave aside to cool down a bit and drizzle over French toasts.

Nutrition Value:
calories 207, fat 15, fiber 1, carbs 1, protein 9

Easy Pancakes

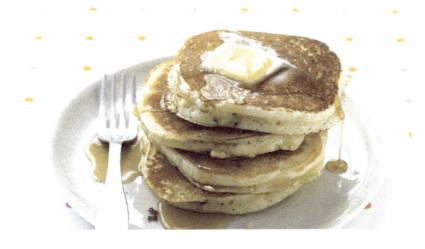

Servings: 4
Prep time: 10 min

INGREDIENTS:

½ teaspoon cinnamon, ground
1 teaspoon stevia
2 eggs
Cooking spray
2 ounces cream cheese

DESCRIPTION:

In a blender, mix eggs with cream cheese, stevia and
cinnamon.

Heat a pan with cooking spray and pour in ¼ of the batter, spread well, cook for 2 minutes, flip and cook for about 2 minutes more.
Transfer to a tray and repeat the action with the rest of the batter.
Serve immediately.

Nutrition Value:
calories 346, fat 27, fiber 12, carbs 3, protein 19

Brussels Sprouts Delight

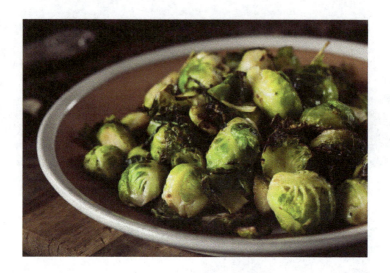

Servings: 4
Prep time: 10 min

INGREDIENTS:

3 eggs
Salt and black pepper to the taste
1 tablespoon ghee, melted
2 shallots, minced
2 garlic cloves, minced
12 ounces Brussels sprouts, thinly sliced
2 ounces bacon, chopped
1 and ½ tablespoons apple cider vinegar

DESCRIPTION:

Warm-up a pan over medium heat, add bacon, stir, cook until it's crispy, transfer to a plate and leave aside for now.

Heat up the pan again over medium heat, add shallots and garlic, stir, and cook for 30 seconds.

Add Brussels sprouts, salt, pepper, and apple cider vinegar, stir and cook for 5 minutes.

Return bacon to pan, stir and cook for 5 minutes more.

Add ghee, stir and make a hole in the center.

Crack eggs into the pan, cook until they are done and serve right away.

Nutrition Value:
calories 248, fat 3, fiber 4, carbs 7, protein 15

Easy Turkey Breakfast

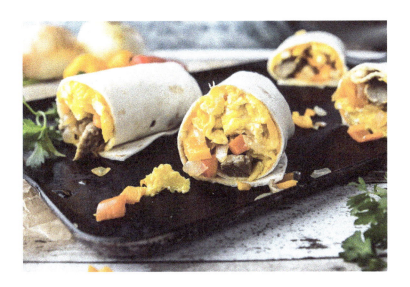

Servings: 4
Prep time: 10 min

INGREDIENTS:

2 avocado slices
Salt and black pepper
2 bacon sliced
2 turkey breast slices, already cooked
2 tablespoons coconut oil
2 eggs, whisked

DESCRIPTION:

Warm up a pan over medium heat, add bacon slices and brown them for a few minutes.

Meanwhile, heat up another pan with the oil over medium heat, add eggs, salt and pepper and scramble them.

Divide turkey breast slices on 2 plates.

Divide scrambled eggs on each.

Divide bacon slices and avocado slices as well and serve.

Nutrition Value:
calories 139, fat 7, fiber 2, carbs 4, protein 16

Easy Breakfast Patties

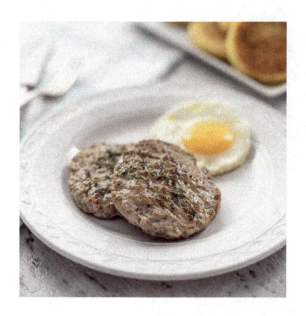

Servings: 4
Prep time: 10 min

INGREDIENTS:

1 pound pork meat, minced
Salt and black pepper to the taste
¼ teaspoon thyme, dried
½ teaspoon sage, dried
¼ teaspoon ginger, dried
3 tablespoon cold water
1 tablespoon coconut oil

DESCRIPTION:

Put meat in a bowl.
In another bowl, mix water with salt, pepper, sage, thyme and ginger and whisk well.
Add this to meat and stir very well.
Shape your patties and place them on a working surface.
Heat up a pan with the coconut oil over medium high heat, add patties, fry them for 5 minutes, flip and cook them for 3 minutes more.
Serve them warm.

Nutrition Value:
calories 324, fat 13, fiber 2, carbs 10, protein 15

Eggs Baked In Avocados

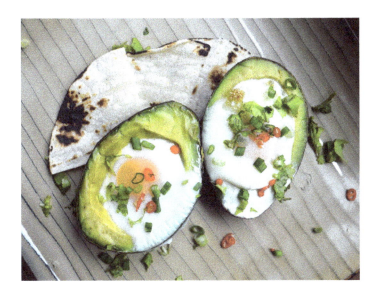

Servings: 4
Prep time: 20 min

INGREDIENTS:

2 avocados, cut in halves and pitted
4 eggs
Salt and black pepper to the taste
1 tablespoon chives, chopped

DESCRIPTION:

Scoop some flesh from the avocado halves and arrange them in a baking dish.
Crack an egg in each avocado, season with salt and pepper, introduce them in the oven at 425 degrees F and bake for 20 minutes.
Sprinkle chives at the end and serve for breakfast!

Nutrition Value:
calories 397, fat 34, fiber 13, carbs 13, protein 15

EASY MEALS

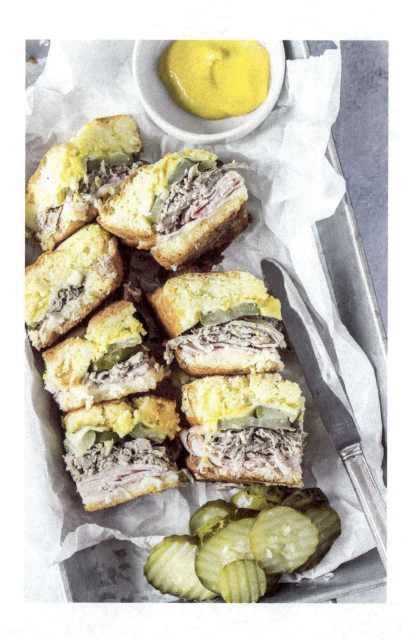

Easy Sausage Salad

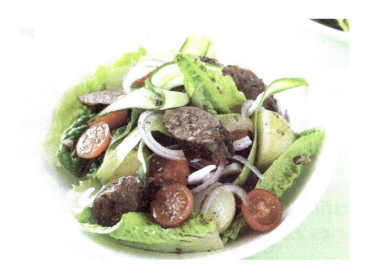

Servings: 4
Prep time: 10 min

INGREDIENTS:

8 pork sausage links, sliced
1 pound cherry tomatoes
4 cups baby spinach
1 tablespoon avocado oil
1 pound mozzarella cheese, cubed
2 tablespoons lemon juice
2/3 cup basil pesto
Salt and black pepper to the taste

DESCRIPTION:

Heat up a pan with the oil over medium high heat, add sausage slices, stir and cook them for 4 minutes on each side.

Meanwhile, in a salad bowl, mix spinach with mozzarella, tomatoes, salt, pepper, lemon juice and pesto and toss to coat.

Add sausage pieces, toss again and serve.

Nutrition Value:
calories 254, fat 16, fiber 3, carbs 8, protein 15

Keto Chili

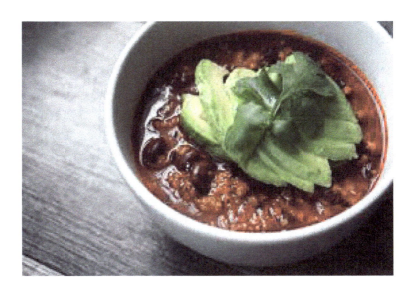

Servings: 8
Prep time: 20 min

INGREDIENTS:

3 slices of bacon (cut into ½-inch strips)
2 chopped celery stalks
1/4 chopped medium yellow onion
1/2 cup sliced baby Bellas
1 chopped green bell pepper
2 pounds ground beef
2 minced cloves garlic
2 teaspoons ground cumin
2 tablespoons chili powder

2 tablespoons smoked paprika
2 teaspoons dried oregano
Kosher salt
Freshly ground black pepper
2 cups low-sodium beef broth
For garnish:
Shredded cheddar
Sour cream
Sliced green onions
Sliced avocado

DESCRIPTION:

Cook bacon in a large pot on moderate heat until crisp. Remove from pot immediately using a slotted spoon and drain on paper towel.
Stir-fry the onion, mushrooms, celery and pepper in the same pot and cook for six minutes until the vegetables are cooked.
Stir in garlic and cook for 1 minute until fragrant.
Push the veggies to the side of pan and place the beef in the center.
Stir and cook until there is no more pink color in the beef.
Drain excess fat from beef and return pan to the heat.
Pour the paprika, oregano, cumin, chili powder, salt and pepper into the beef mixture, stirring often and cook for two minutes.

Pour the broth and simmer; cook for ten to fifteen minutes until the broth is almost dried.
Spoon the chili into individual bowls.
Garnish with sour cream, bacon crisps, shredded cheese, avocado slices and green onions.

Nutrition Value:
calories 234, fat 13, fiber 3, carbs 8, protein 11

Taco Stuffed Peppers

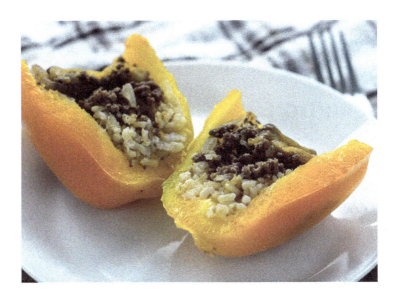

Servings: 8
Prep time: 20 min

INGREDIENTS:

1 pound ground beef
Extra-virgin olive oil
1 minced clove garlic
1/2 chopped onion
Freshly ground black pepper
Kosher salt
1 teaspoon chili powder
2 tablespoons chopped cilantro

1/2 teaspoon smoked paprika
1/2 teaspoon ground cumin
1 cup shredded cheddar
3 bell peppers
1 cup shredded lettuce
1 cup shredded Monterey Jack

DESCRIPTION:

Remove seeds of peppers and cut into half.
Preheat the oven at 375° and coat a large baking dish
with cooking spray.
Heat 1 tablespoon of extra-virgin olive oil in a large
skillet on medium heat.
Sauté the onion and cook for five minutes until
tender. Add the garlic and stir-fry until aromatic for 1
minute longer.
Add beef and stir-fry for five minutes until the
pinkish color is gone; drain excess fat.
Stir in ground cumin, paprika and chili powder and
sprinkle with salt and pepper.
Drizzle the bell peppers with olive oil; season bell
peppers with salt and pepper.
Neatly place the bell peppers with cut side up on the
baking dish.
Stuff each pepper with a meat mixture.
Sprinkle stuffed pepper with cheese, bake for twenty
minutes until tender-crisp and the cheese melts.

Place on top with shredded lettuce. Serve with hot sauce, Pico de Gallo and lime wedges.

Nutrition Value:

244 calorie; 10.2 g fat ;77 mg chol; 282 mg sodium; 8.1 g carbohydrate; 1.6 g dietary fiber; 4 g total sugars; 29.7 g protein.

Keto Burger Fat Bombs

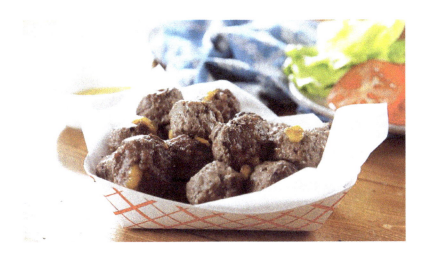

Servings: 8
Prep time: 20 min

INGREDIENTS:
Cooking spray
1 pound ground beef
Kosher salt
1/2 teaspoon garlic powder
2 tablespoons cold butter (cut into 20 pieces)
Freshly ground black pepper
1/4 (8 ounces) block cheddar cheese (cut into 20 pieces)

DESCRIPTION:

Preheat oven at 375° F.
Prepare a mini muffin tin by greasing with cooking spray.
Combine in a medium-sized bowl the beef with salt, pepper and garlic powder.
Spoon 1 tablespoon of beef mixture and press into the bottom of muffin tin cup.
Put one piece of butter on top of meat and then press 1 tablespoon of beef mixture on top of butter.
Put on top of meat one piece of cheese and put another beef on top of cheese to cover.
Do these steps for the rest of beef, butter, beef, cheese, and beef for the rest of muffin tin cups.
Bake for fifteen minutes until the meat is no longer pinkish in color, let cool slightly before removing from tin with a metal offset spatula.
Serve Keto burgers with lettuce leaves, ripe tomatoes and mustard.

Nutrition Value:
99 calorie; 6.2 g fat; 35 mg cholesterol; 104 mg sodium; 0.9 g carbohydrate; 0.2 g dietary fiber; ; 9.8 g protein.

Cheese Taco Shells

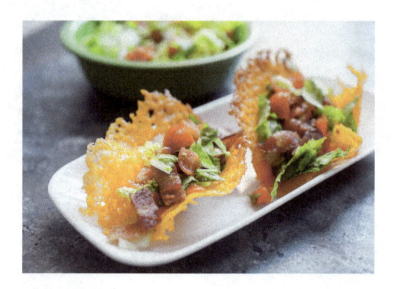

Servings: 6
Prep time: 20 min

INGREDIENTS:

1 pound ground beef
2 cups shredded cheddar
1 tablespoons vegetable oil
Freshly ground black pepper
1 tablespoon taco seasoning
1 chopped white onion

DESCRIPTION:

Preheat oven at 375 degrees F. Place parchment paper on the baking sheet and spray on top with cooking spray.

Spoon about ½ cup of cheddar mound and place on the baking sheet; season with pepper.

Bake until the cheese is becoming melty and a bit crispy for five to seven minutes.

Turn upside down two drinking glasses and connect the two glasses with a wooden spoon to resemble like a bridge.

With a spatula, hang the cheese mounds on the wooden spoon to create taco shells. Let cool.

Heat the vegetable oil in a large skillet on moderate heat.

Cook the onions for five minutes until soft and stir in ground beef until brownish for six minutes longer. Drain excess fats. Stir in taco seasoning.

To assemble, fill each cheese taco with sautéed beef and garnish with shredded lettuce and chopped tomatoes. Serve with hot sauce.

Nutrition Value:
365 calorie; 14.5 g fat; 113 mg cholesterol; 686 mg sodium; 6.9 g carbohydrate; 1 g diet fiber; 48.7 g protein.

Veal Parmesan

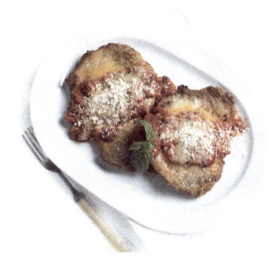

Servings: 4
Prep time: 40 min

INGREDIENTS:

8 veal cutlets
2/3 cup parmesan, grated
8 provolone cheese slices
Salt and black pepper to the taste
5 cups tomato sauce
A pinch of garlic salt
Cooking spray
2 tablespoons ghee
2 tablespoons coconut oil, melted

1 teaspoon Italian seasoning

DESCRIPTION:

Season veal cutlets with salt, pepper and garlic salt,
Heat up a pan with the ghee and the oil over medium
high heat, add veal and cook until they brown on all
sides.
Spread half of the tomato sauce on the bottom of a
baking dish which you've greased with some cooking
spray.
Add veal cutlets, then sprinkle Italian seasoning and
spread the rest of the sauce.
Cover dish, introduce in the oven at 350 degrees F
and bake for 40 minutes.
Uncover dish, spread provolone cheese and sprinkle
parmesan, introduce in the oven again and bake for
15 minutes more.
Divide between plates and serve.

Nutrition Value:
**calories 366, fat 25, fiber 2, carbs 6, protein
26**

Roasted Beef

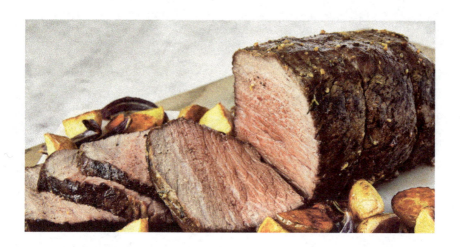

Servings: 4
Prep time: 40 min

INGREDIENTS:

5 pounds beef roast
Salt and black pepper to the taste
½ teaspoon celery salt
2 teaspoons chili powder
1 tablespoon avocado oil
1 tablespoon sweet paprika
A pinch of cayenne pepper
½ teaspoon garlic powder
½ cup beef stock
1 tablespoon garlic, minced

¼ teaspoon dry mustard

DESCRIPTION:

Warm-up a pan with the oil over medium-high heat, add beef roast and brown it on all sides.
In a bowl, mix paprika with chili powder, celery salt, salt, pepper, cayenne, garlic powder and mustard powder and stir.
Add roast, rub well and transfer it to a Crockpot.
Add beef stock and garlic over roast and cook on Low for 8 hours.
Transfer beef to a cutting board, leave it to cool down a bit, slice and divide between plates.
Strain juices from the pot, drizzle over meat and serve.

Nutrition Value:
calories 185, fat 5, fiber 1, carbs 5, protein 23

Amazing Tilapia

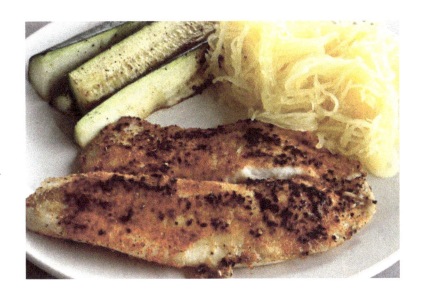

Servings: 4
Prep time: 40 min

INGREDIENTS:

4 tilapia fillets, boneless
Salt and black pepper to the taste
½ cup parmesan, grated
4 tablespoons mayonnaise
¼ teaspoon basil, dried
¼ teaspoon garlic powder
2 tablespoons lemon juice
¼ cup ghee

Cooking spray
A pinch of onion powder

DESCRIPTION:

Spray a baking sheet, place tilapia on it, season with salt and pepper, introduce in preheated broiler and cook for 4 minutes.
Turn fish on the other side and broil for 4 minutes more.
In a bowl, mix parmesan with mayo, basil, garlic, lemon juice, onion powder and ghee and stir well.
Add fish to this mix, toss to coat well, place on the baking sheet again and broil for 3 minutes more.
Transfer to plates and serve.

Nutrition Value:
calories 185, fat 10, fiber 0, carbs 2, protein 15

Trout And Ghee Sauce

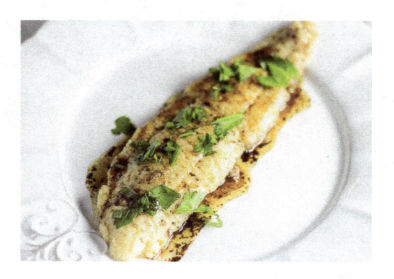

Servings: 4
Prep time: 40 min

INGREDIENTS:

4 trout fillets
Salt and black pepper to the taste
3 teaspoons lemon zest, grated
3 tablespoons chives, chopped
6 tablespoons ghee
2 tablespoons olive oil
2 teaspoons lemon juice

DESCRIPTION:

Season trout with salt and pepper, drizzle the olive oil
and massage a bit.
Heat up your kitchen grill over medium high heat,
add fish fillets, cook for 4 minutes, flip and cook for 4
minutes more.
Meanwhile, heat up a pan with the ghee over medium
heat, add salt, pepper, chives, lemon juice and zest
and stir well.
Divide fish fillets on plates, drizzle the ghee sauce
over them and serve.

Nutrition Value:
calories 324, fat 14, fiber 1, carbs 2, protein 25

Baked Halibut

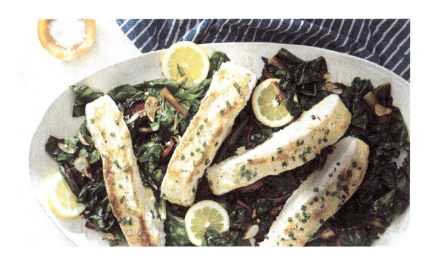

Servings: 4
Prep time: 10 min

INGREDIENTS:

½ cup parmesan, grated
¼ cup ghee
¼ cup mayonnaise
2 tablespoons green onions, chopped
6 garlic cloves, minced
A dash of Tabasco sauce
4 halibut fillets
Salt and black pepper to the taste

Juice of ½ lemon

DESCRIPTION:

Season halibut with salt, pepper and some of the lemon juice, place in a baking dish and cook in the oven at 450 degrees F for 6 minutes.
Meanwhile, heat up a pan with the ghee over medium heat, add parmesan, mayo, green onions, Tabasco sauce, garlic and the rest of the lemon juice and stir well.
Take fish out of the oven, drizzle parmesan sauce all over, turn oven to broil and broil your fish for 3 minutes.
Divide between plates and serve.

Nutrition Value:
calories 246, fat 12, fiber 1, carbs 5, protein 22

Crusted Salmon

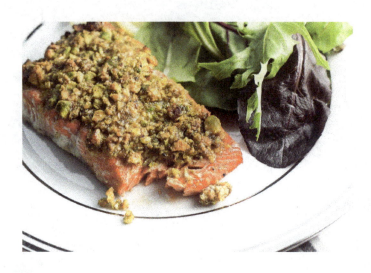

Servings: 4
Prep time: 15 min

INGREDIENTS:

3 garlic cloves, minced
2 pounds salmon fillet
Salt and black pepper to the taste
½ cup parmesan, grated
¼ cup parsley, chopped

DESCRIPTION:

Put salmon on a lined baking sheet, season with salt and pepper, cover with a parchment paper, introduce in the oven at 425 degrees F and bake for 10 minutes. Take fish out of the oven, sprinkle parmesan, parsley and garlic over fish, introduce in the oven again and cook for 5 minutes more.
Divide between plates and serve.

Nutrition Value:
calories 244, fat 12, fiber 1, carbs 0.6, protein 20

Very Tasty Cod

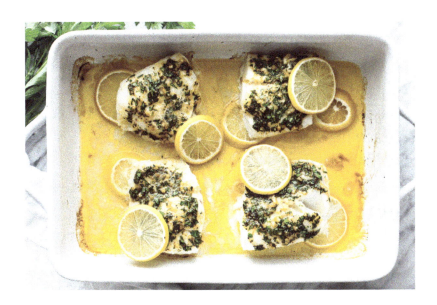

Servings: 4
Prep time: 20 min

INGREDIENTS:

1 pound cod, cut into medium pieces
Salt and black pepper to the taste
2 green onions, chopped
3 garlic cloves, minced
3 tablespoons soy sauce
1 cup fish stock
1 tablespoon balsamic vinegar
1 tablespoon ginger, grated

½ teaspoon chili pepper, crushed

DESCRIPTION:

Warm-up a pan over medium-high heat, add fish
pieces andbrown it a few minutes on each side.
Add garlic, green onions, salt, pepper, soy sauce, fish
stock, vinegar, chili pepper and ginger stir, cover,
reduce heat and cook for 20 minutes.
Divide between plates and serve.

Nutrition Value:
calories 158, fat 3, fiber 2, carbs 4, protein 21

Cod With Arugula

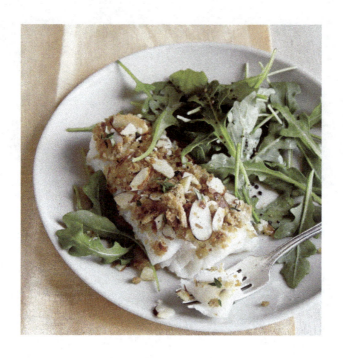

Servings: 4
Prep time: 20 min

INGREDIENTS:

2 cod fillets
1 tablespoon olive oil
Salt and black pepper to the taste
Juice of 1 lemon
3 cup arugula
½ cup black olives, pitted and sliced

2 tablespoons capers
1 garlic clove, chopped

DESCRIPTION:

Arrange fish fillets in a heatproof dish, season with salt, pepper, drizzle the oil and lemon juice, toss to coat, introduce in the oven at 450 degrees F and bake for 20 minutes.
In your food processor, mix arugula with salt, pepper, capers, olives and garlic and blend a bit.
Arrange fish on plates, top with arugula tapenade and serve.

Nutrition Value:
calories 241, fat 5, fiber 3, carbs 3, protein 14

Tasty Fish Curry

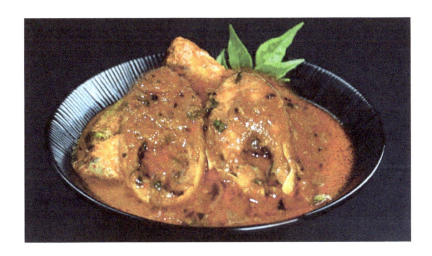

Servings: 6
Prep time: 25 min

INGREDIENTS:

4 white fish fillets
½ teaspoon mustard seeds
Salt and black pepper to the taste
2 green chilies, chopped
1 teaspoon ginger, grated
1 teaspoon curry powder
¼ teaspoon cumin, ground
4 tablespoons coconut oil
1 small red onion, chopped
1-inch turmeric root, grated

¼ cup cilantro
1 and ½ cups coconut cream
3 garlic cloves, minced

DESCRIPTION:

Heat up a pot with half of the coconut oil over
medium heat, add mustard seeds and cook for 2
minutes. Add ginger, onion, and garlic, stir and cook
for 5 minutes.
Add turmeric, curry powder, chilies, and cumin stir
and cook for 5 minutes more.
Add coconut milk, salt, and pepper, stir, bring to a
boil and cook for 15 minutes.
Heat up another pan with the rest of the oil over
medium heat, add fish, stir and cook for 3 minutes.
Add this to the curry sauce, stir and cook for 5
minutes more.
Add cilantro, stir, divide into bowls and serve.

Nutrition Value:
**calories 504, fat 34, fiber 7, carbs 6, protein
48**

Delicious Easy Shrimp

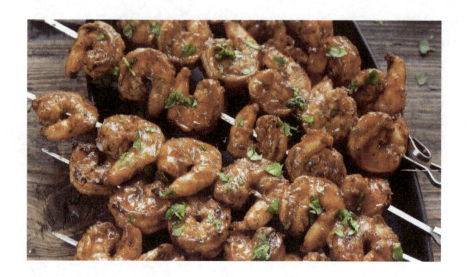

Servings: 4
Prep time: 10 min

INGREDIENTS:

2 tablespoons olive oil
1 tablespoon ghee
1 pound shrimp, peeled and deveined
2 tablespoons lemon juice
2 tablespoons garlic, minced
1 tablespoon lemon zest
Salt and black pepper to the taste

DESCRIPTION:

Warm-up a pan with the oil and the ghee over medium-high heat, add shrimp and cook for 2 minutes.
Add garlic, stir and cook for 4 minutes more.
Add lemon juice, lemon zest, salt and pepper, stir, take off heat and serve.

Nutrition Value:
calories 159, fat 1, fiber 3, carbs 1, protein 4

Shrimp And Noodle Salad

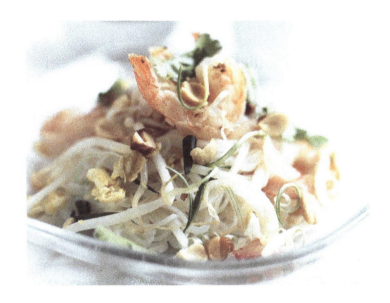

Servings: 4
Prep time: 10 min

INGREDIENTS:

1 cucumber, cut with a spiralizer
½ cup basil, chopped
½ pound shrimp, already cooked, peeled and deveined
Salt and black pepper to the taste
1 tablespoon stevia
2 teaspoons fish sauce

2 tablespoons lime juice
2 teaspoons chili garlic sauce

DESCRIPTION:

Put cucumber noodles on a paper towel, cover with
another one and press well.
Put into a bowl and mix with basil, shrimp, salt and
pepper.
In another bowl, mix stevia with fish sauce, lime juice
and chili sauce and whisk well.
Add this to shrimp salad, toss to coat well and serve.

Nutrition Value:
calories 135, fat 2, fiber 3, carbs 1, protein 8

Easy Spicy Shrimp

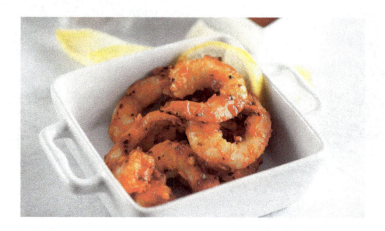

Servings: 4
Prep time: 8 min

INGREDIENTS:

½ pound big shrimp, peeled and deveined
2 teaspoons Worcestershire sauce
2 teaspoons olive oil
Juice of 1 lemon
Salt and black pepper to the taste
1 teaspoon Creole seasoning

DESCRIPTION:

Arrange shrimp in one layer in a baking dish, season
with salt and pepper and drizzle the oil.

Add Worcestershire sauce, lemon juice and sprinkle Creole seasoning.
Toss shrimp a bit, introduce in the oven, set it on the broiler and cook for 8 minutes.
Divide between 2 plates and serve.

Nutrition Value:
calories 124, fat 3, fiber 1, carbs 2, protein 9

Simple Mussels Dish

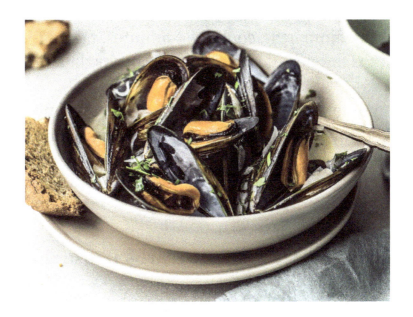

Servings: 4
Prep time: 8 min

INGREDIENTS:

2 pound mussels, debearded and scrubbed
2 garlic cloves, minced
1 tablespoon ghee
A splash of lemon juice

DESCRIPTION:

Put some water in a pot, add mussels, bring to a boil over medium heat, cook for 5 minutes, take off heat, discard unopened mussels and transfer them to a bowl.
In another bowl, mix ghee with garlic and lemon juice, whisk and heat up in the microwave for 1 minute.
Pour over mussels and serve them right away.

Nutrition Value:
calories 56, fat 1, fiber 0, carbs 1, protein 2

Calamari Salad

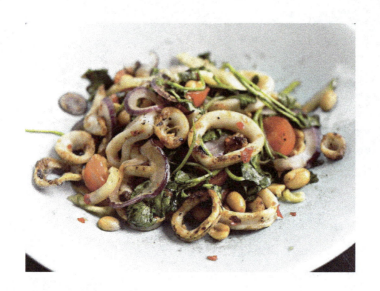

Servings: 4
Prep time: 30 min

INGREDIENTS:

2 long red chilies, chopped
2 small red chilies, chopped
2 garlic cloves, minced
3 green onions, chopped
1 tablespoon balsamic vinegar
Salt and black pepper to the taste
Juice of 1 lemon
6 pounds calamari hoods, tentacles reserved
3.5 ounces olive oil

3 ounces rocket for serving

DESCRIPTION:

In a bowl, mix long red chilies with small red chilies, green onions, vinegar, half of the oil, garlic, salt, pepper and lemon juice and stir well.
Place calamari and tentacles in a bowl, season with salt and pepper, drizzle the rest of the oil, toss to coat and place on preheated grill over medium high heat.
Cook for few minutes on each side and transfer to the chili marinade you've made.
Toss to coat and leave aside for 30 minutes.
Arrange rocket on plates, top with calamari and its marinade and serve.

Nutrition Value:
calories 210, fat 4, fiber 2, carbs 2, protein 4

Swiss Chard Salad

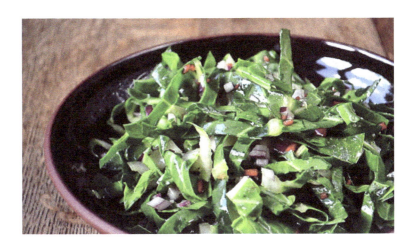

Servings: 4
Prep time: 30 min

INGREDIENTS:

2 bunch Swiss chard, cut into strips 2 tablespoons avocado oil
1 small yellow onion, chopped A pinch of red pepper flakes
¼ cup pine nuts, toasted
¼ cup raisins
1 tablespoon balsamic vinegar Salt and black pepper to the taste

DESCRIPTION:

Heat up a pan with the oil over medium heat, add chard and onions, stir and cook for 5 minutes.
Add salt, pepper and pepper flakes, stir and cook for 3 minutes more.
Put raisins in a bowl, add water to cover them, heat them up in your microwave for 1 minute, leave aside for 5 minutes and drain them well.
Add raisins and pine nuts to the pan, also add vinegar, stir, cook for 3 minutes more, divide between plates and serve.

NutritionValue:
calories 125, fat 2, fiber 1, carbs 4, protein 5

Catalan Style Greens

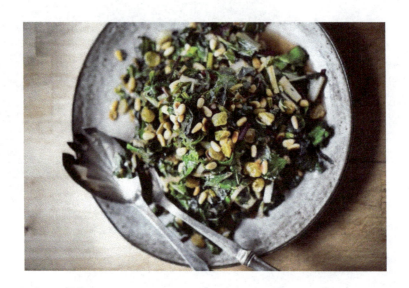

Servings: 4
Prep time: 30 min

INGREDIENTS:

1 apple, cored and chopped
1 yellow onion, sliced
3 tablespoons avocado oil
¼ cup raisins
6 garlic cloves, chopped
¼ cup pine nuts, toasted
¼ cup balsamic vinegar
5 cups mixed spinach and chard
Salt and black pepper to the taste

A pinch of nutmeg

DESCRIPTION:

Warm-up a pan with the oil over medium-high heat, add onion, stir and cook for 3 minutes.
Add apple, stir and cook for 4 minutes more.
Add garlic, stir and cook for 1 minute.
Add raisins, vinegar and mixed spinach and chard, stir and cook for 5 minutes.
Add nutmeg, salt and pepper, stir, cook for a few seconds more, divide between plates and serve.

Nutrition Value:
calories 124, fat 1, fiber 2, carbs 3, protein 9

Swiss Chard Soup

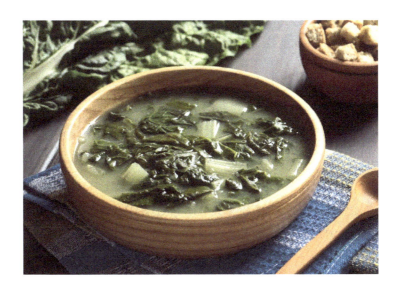

Servings: 8
Prep time: 35 min

INGREDIENTS:

4 cups Swiss chard, chopped
4 cups chicken breast, cooked and shredded
2 cups water
1 cup mushrooms, sliced
1 tablespoon garlic, minced
1 tablespoon coconut oil, melted
¼ cup onion, chopped
8 cups chicken stock

2 cups yellow squash, chopped
1 cup green beans, cut into medium pieces
2 tablespoons vinegar
¼ cup basil, chopped
Salt and black pepper to the taste
4 bacon slices, chopped
¼ cup sundried tomatoes, chopped

DESCRIPTION:

Heat up a pot with the oil over medium-high heat, add bacon, stir and cook for 2 minutes.
Add tomatoes, garlic, onions and mushrooms, stir and cook for 5 minutes.
Add water, stock and chicken, stir and cook for 15 minutes.
Add Swiss chard, green beans, squash, salt and pepper, stir and cook for 10 minutes more.
Add vinegar, basil, more salt and pepper if needed, stir, ladle into soup bowls and serve.

Nutrition Value:
calories 144, fat 4, fiber 2, carbs 4, protein 15

Easy Cabbage Soup

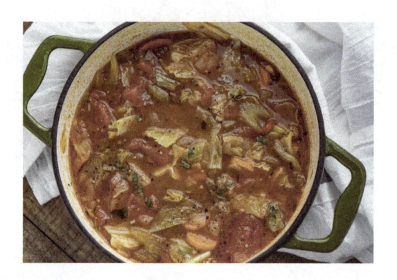

Servings: 6
Prep time: 45 min

INGREDIENTS:

1 garlic clove, minced
1 cabbage head, chopped
2 pounds beef, ground
1 yellow onion, chopped
1 teaspoon cumin
4 bouillon cubes
Salt and black pepper to the taste
10 ounces canned tomatoes and green chilies
4 cups water

DESCRIPTION:

Warm-up a pan over medium heat, add beef, stir and brown for a few minutes.

Add onion, stir, cook for 4 minutes more and transfer to a pot.

Heat up, add cabbage, cumin, garlic, bouillon cubes, tomatoes and chilies and water, stir, bring to a boil over high heat, cover, reduce temperature and cook for 40 minutes.

Season with salt and pepper, stir, ladle into soup bowls and serve.

Nutrition Value:
calories 206, fat 3, fiber 2, carbs 3, protein 4

Arugula Soup

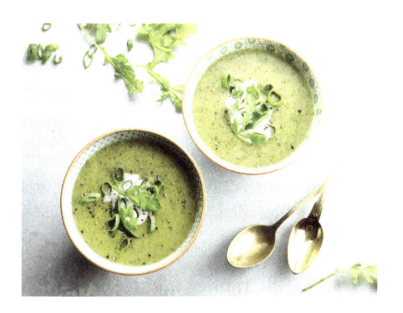

Servings: 6
Prep time: 15 min

INGREDIENTS:

1 yellow onion, chopped
1 tablespoon olive oil
2 garlic cloves, minced
½ cup coconut milk
10 ounces baby arugula
¼ cup mixed mint, tarragon and parsley
2 tablespoons chives, chopped
4 tablespoons coconut milk yogurt

6 cups chicken stock
Salt and black pepper to the taste

DESCRIPTION:

Heat up a pot with the oil over medium high heat, add onion and garlic, stir and cook for 5 minutes.
Add stock and milk, stir and bring to a simmer.
Add arugula, tarragon, parsley and mint, stir and cook everything for 6 minutes.
Add coconut yogurt, salt, pepper and chives, stir, cook for 2 minutes, divide into soup bowls and serve.

Nutrition Value:
calories 210, fat 4, fiber 2, carbs 6, protein 9

Thai Avocado Soup

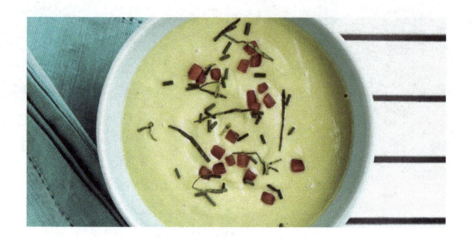

Servings: 6
Prep time: 15 min

INGREDIENTS:

1 cup coconut milk
2 teaspoons Thai green curry paste
1 avocado, pitted, peeled and chopped
1 tablespoon cilantro, chopped
Salt and black pepper to the taste
2 cups veggie stock
Lime wedges for serving

DESCRIPTION:

In your blender, mix avocado with salt, pepper, curry paste and coconut milk and pulse well.
Transfer this to a pot and heat up over medium heat.
Add stock, stir, bring to a simmer and cook for 5 minutes.
Add cilantro, more salt and pepper, stir, cook for 2 minute more, ladle into soup bowls and serve with lime wedges on the side.

Nutrition Value:
calories 245, fat 4, fiber 3, carbs 6, protein 18

Avocado And Egg Salad

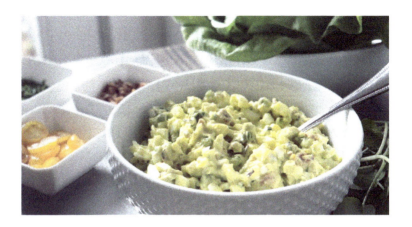

Servings: 4
Prep time: 8 min

INGREDIENTS:

4 cups mixed lettuce leaves, torn
4 eggs
1 avocado, pitted and sliced
¼ cup mayonnaise
2 teaspoons mustard
2 garlic cloves, minced
1 tablespoon chives, chopped
Salt and black pepper to the taste

DESCRIPTION:

Put the water in a pot, add some salt, add eggs, bring
to a boilover medium-high heat, boil for 7 minutes,
drain, cool, peel and chop them.
In a salad bowl, mix lettuce with eggs and avocado.
Add chives and garlic, some salt and pepper and toss
to coat.
In a bowl, mix mustard with mayo, salt and pepper
and stir well.
Add this to salad, toss well and serve right away.

Nutrition Value:
calories 237, fat 12, fiber 4, carbs 9, protein 16

Creamy Radishes

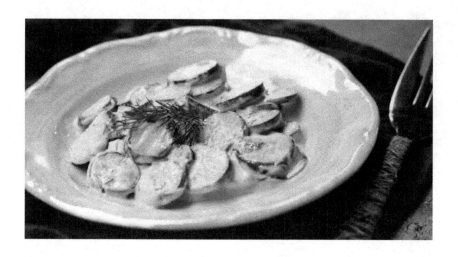

Servings: 4
Prep time: 25 min

INGREDIENTS:

7 ounces radishes, cut in halves
2 tablespoons sour cream
2 bacon slices
1 tablespoon green onion, chopped
1 tablespoon cheddar cheese, grated
Hot sauce to the taste
Salt and black pepper to the taste

DESCRIPTION:

Put radishes into a pot, add water to cover, bring to a boil over medium heat, cook them for 10 minutes and drain.

Heat up a pan over medium high heat, add bacon, cook until it's crispy, transfer to paper towels, drain grease, crumble and leave aside.

Return pan to medium heat, add radishes, stir and sauté them for 7 minutes.

Add onion, salt, pepper, hot sauce and sour cream, stir and cook for 7 minutes more.

Transfer to a plate, top with crumbled bacon and cheddar cheese and serve.

Nutrition Value:
calories 344, fat 23, fiber 3, carbs 6, protein 12

Roasted Radishes

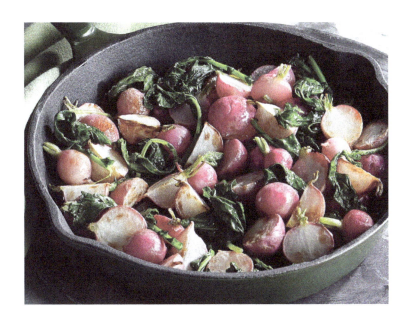

Servings: 4
Prep time: 35 min

INGREDIENTS:

2 cups radishes, cut in quarters
Salt and black pepper to the taste
2 tablespoons ghee, melted
1 tablespoon chives, chopped
1 tablespoon lemon zest

DESCRIPTION:

Spread radishes on a lined baking sheet.
Add salt and pepper, chives, lemon zest and ghee,
toss to coat and bake in the oven at 375 F for 35
minutes.
Divide between plates and serve.

Nutrition Value:
calories 126, fat 12, fiber 1, carbs 5, protein 12

Asparagus Frittata

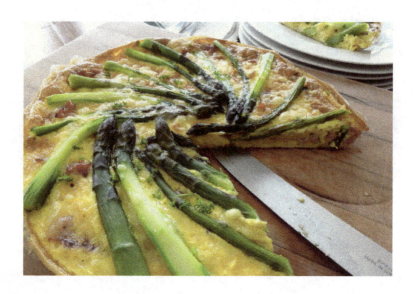

Servings: 4
Prep time: 10 min

INGREDIENTS:

¼ cup yellow onion, chopped
A drizzle of olive oil
1 pound asparagus spears, cut into 1 inch pieces
Salt and black pepper to the taste
4 eggs, whisked
1 cup cheddar cheese, grated

DESCRIPTION:

Heat up a pan with the oil over medium high heat, add onions, stir and cook for 3 minutes.
Add asparagus, stir and cook for 6 minutes.
Add eggs, stir a bit and cook for 3 minutes.
Add salt, pepper and sprinkle the cheese, introduce in the oven and broil for 3 minutes.
Divide frittata between plates and serve.

Nutrition Value:
calories 205, fat 12, fiber 2, carbs 8, protein 14

Cream Of Celery

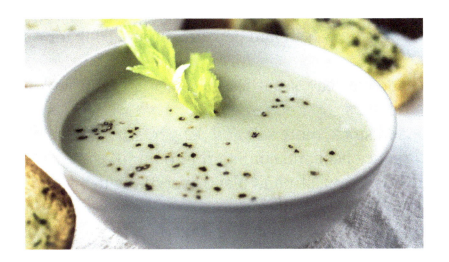

Servings: 4
Prep time: 10 min

INGREDIENTS:

1 bunch celery, chopped
Salt and black pepper to the taste
3 bay leaves
½ garlic head, chopped
2 yellow onions, chopped
4 cups chicken stock
¾ cup heavy cream
2 tablespoons ghee

DESCRIPTION:

Warm-up a pot with the ghee over medium-high heat, add onions, salt and pepper, stir and cook for 5 minutes.
Add bay leaves, garlic and celery, stir and cook for 15 minutes.
Add stock, more salt and pepper, stir, cover pot, reduce heat and simmer for 20 minutes.
Add cream, stir and blend everything using an immersion blender.
Ladle into soup bowls and serve.

Nutrition Value:
calories 156, fat 3, fiber 1, carbs 2, protein 9

Delicious Whole Chicken

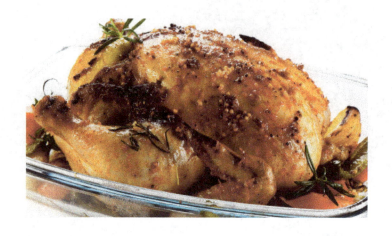

Servings: 4
Prep time: 40 min

INGREDIENTS:

1 whole chicken
½ teaspoon onion powder
½ teaspoon garlic powder
Salt and black pepper to the taste
2 tablespoons coconut oil
1 teaspoon Italian seasoning
1 and ½ cups chicken stock
2 teaspoons guar guar

DESCRIPTION:

Rub chicken with half of the oil, garlic powder, salt, pepper, Italian seasoning and onion powder.
Put the rest of the oil into an instant pot and add chicken to the pot.
Add stock, cover pot and cook on High for 40 minutes.
Transfer chicken to a platter and leave aside for now.
Set the instant pot on Sauté mode, add guar guar, stir and cook until it thickens.
Pour sauce over chicken and serve.

Nutrition Value:
calories 448, fat 30, fiber 1, carbs 1, protein 38

Easy Balsamic Chicken

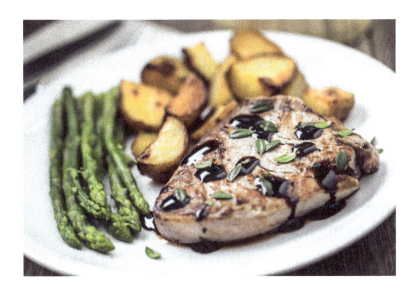

Servings: 4
Prep time: 40 min

INGREDIENTS:

3 tablespoons coconut oil
2 pounds chicken breasts, skinless and boneless
3 garlic cloves, minced
Salt and black pepper to the taste
1 cup chicken stock
3 tablespoons stevia
½ cup balsamic vinegar
1 tomato, thinly sliced

6 mozzarella slices
Some chopped basil for serving

DESCRIPTION:

Heat up a pan with the oil over medium high heat,
add chicken pieces, season with salt and pepper, cook
until they brown on both sides and reduce heat.
Add garlic, vinegar, stock and stevia, stir, increase
heat again and cook for 10 minutes.
Transfer chicken breasts to a lined baking sheet,
arrange mozzarella slices on top, then top with basil.
Broil in the oven over medium heat until cheese melts
and then arrange tomato slices over chicken pieces.
Divide between plates and serve.

Nutrition Value:
calories 244, fat 12, fiber 1, carbs 6, protein 29

Jamaican Pork

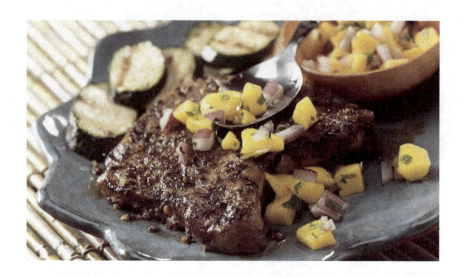

Servings: 4
Prep time: 40 min

INGREDIENTS:

4 pounds pork shoulder
1 tablespoon coconut oil
½ cup beef stock
¼ cup Jamaican jerk spice mix

DESCRIPTION:

Rub pork shoulder with Jamaican mix and place in
your instant pot.

Add oil to the pot and set it to Sauté mode.
Add pork shoulder and brown it on all sides.
Add stock, cover pot and cook on High for 45
minutes.
Uncover pot, transfer pork to a platter, shred and
serve.

Nutrition Value:
**calories 254, fat 20, fiber 0, carbs 0, protein
22**

Juicy Pork Chops

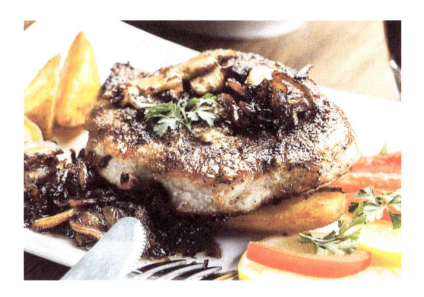

Servings: 4
Prep time: 40 min

INGREDIENTS:

2 yellow onions, chopped
6 bacon slices, chopped
½ cup chicken stock
Salt and black pepper to the taste
4 pork chops

DESCRIPTION:

Warm-up a pan over medium heat, add bacon, stir, cook until it's crispy and transfer to a bowl.
Return pan to medium heat, add onions, some salt, and pepper,stir, cover, cook for 15 minutes and transfer to the same bowl with the bacon.
Return pan once again to heat, increase to medium-high, add pork chop, season with salt and pepper, brown for 3 minutes on one side, flip, reduce heat to medium, and cook for 7 minutes more.
Add stock, stir and cook for 2 minutes more.
Return bacon and onions to the pan, stir, cook for 1 minute more, divide between plates and serve.

Nutrition Value:
calories 328, fat 18, fiber 1, carbs 6, protein 31

Simple Asparagus Fries

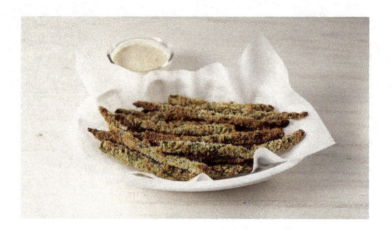

Servings: 4
Prep time: 10 min

INGREDIENTS:

¼ cup parmesan, grated
16 asparagus spears, trimmed
1 egg, whisked
½ teaspoon onion powder
2 ounces pork rinds

DESCRIPTION:

Crush pork rinds and put them in a bowl.
Add onion powder and cheese and stir everything.

Roll asparagus spears in egg, then dip them in pork rind mix and arrange them all on a lined baking sheet.

Introduce in the oven at 425 degrees F and bake for 10 minutes.

Divide between plates and serve them with some sour cream on the side.

Nutrition Value:
calories 128, fat 2, fiber 2, carbs 7, protein 9

Crusted Lamb Chops

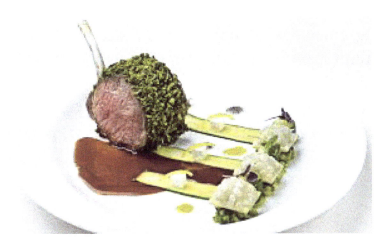

Servings: 4
Prep time: 10 min

INGREDIENTS:

2 lamb racks, cut into chops
Salt and black pepper to the taste
3 tablespoons paprika
¾ cup cumin powder
1 teaspoon chili powder

DESCRIPTION:

In a bowl, mix paprika with cumin, chili, salt and
pepper and stir.

Add lamb chops and rub them well.
Heat up your grill over medium temperature, add lamb chops, cook for 5 minutes, flip and cook for 5 minutes more.
Flip them again, cook for 2 minutes and then for 2 minutes more on the other side again.

Nutrition Value:
calories 204, fat 5, fiber 3, carbs 4, protein 6

Conclusions

The Keto diet is not easy to write about because it is

 often difficult to follow programmatically, but above

all its recipes are very laborious and difficult to

prepare...

I hope that this book has made the whole process

easier.

of preparation, and I hope with all my heart that you

can achieve all your goals....

See you in the next book....

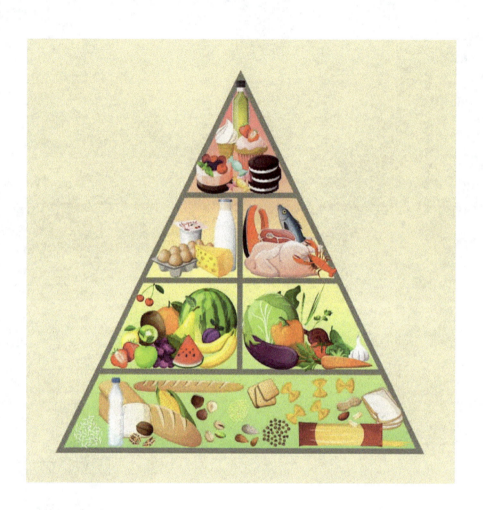

9 781802 863284